The Ultimate M
Recipe Collection

A Complete Collection of Healthy Recipes to Discover
the Benefits of Mediterranean Diet

America Best Recipes

Table of contents

Sorghum Bake

Preparation Time: 10 minutes

Cooking Time: 25 minutes

Servings: 4

Ingredients:

- ½ cup sorghum
- 1 apple, chopped
- 1 oz raisins
- 1.5cup of water

Directions:

1. Put sorghum in the pan. Flatten it.
2. Then top it with raisins, apple, and water.
3. Cover the meal with baking paper and transfer in the preheated to 375F oven.
4. Bake the meal for 25 minutes.

Nutrition:

Calories: 179;

Protein: 18.3g;

Carbs: 3.4g;

Fat: 19.3g

Lamb and Chickpeas Stew

Preparation Time: 10 minutes

Cooking Time: 1 hour and 20 minutes

Servings: 6

Ingredients:

- 1 and ½ lb. lamb shoulder, cubed
- 3 tbsp. olive oil
- 1 cup yellow onion, chopped
- 1 cup carrots, cubed
- 1 cup celery, chopped
- 3 garlic cloves, minced
- 4 rosemary springs, chopped
- 2 cups chicken stock
- 1 cup tomato puree
- 15 oz. canned chickpeas, drained and rinsed
- 10 oz. baby spinach
- 2 tbsp. black olives, pitted and sliced
- A pinch of salt and black pepper

Directions:

1. Heat up a pot with the oil over medium-high heat, add the meat, salt and pepper and brown for 5 minutes.
2. Add carrots, celery, onion and garlic, stir and sauté for 5 minutes more.
3. Add the rosemary, stock, chickpeas and the other ingredients except the spinach and olives, stir and cook for 1 hour.
4. Add the rest of the ingredients, cook the stew over medium heat for 10 minutes more, divide into bowls and serve.

Nutrition: Calories 340, Fat 16gg, Fiber 3g, Carbs 21g, Protein 19g

Chorizo and Lentils Stew

Preparation Time: 10 minutes

Cooking Time: 35 minutes

Servings: 4

Ingredients:

- 4 cups water
- 1 cup carrots, sliced
- 1 yellow onion, chopped
- 1 tbsp. extra-virgin olive oil
- ¾ cup celery, chopped
- 1 and ½ tsp. garlic, minced
- 1 and ½ lb. gold potatoes, roughly chopped
- 7 oz. chorizo, cut in half lengthwise and thinly sliced
- 1 and ½ cup lentils
- ½ tsp. smoked paprika
- ½ tsp. oregano
- Salt and black pepper to taste
- 14 oz. canned tomatoes, chopped
- ½ cup cilantro, chopped

Directions:

1. Heat a saucepan with oil over medium high heat, add onion, garlic, celery and carrots, stir and cook for 4 minutes.
2. Add the chorizo, stir and cook for 1 minute more.
3. Add the rest of the ingredients except the cilantro, stir, bring to a boil, reduce heat to medium-low and simmer for 25 minutes.
4. Divide the stew into bowls and serve with the cilantro sprinkled on top. Enjoy!

Nutrition: Calories 400, Fat 16gg, Fiber 13g, Carbs 58g, Protein 24g

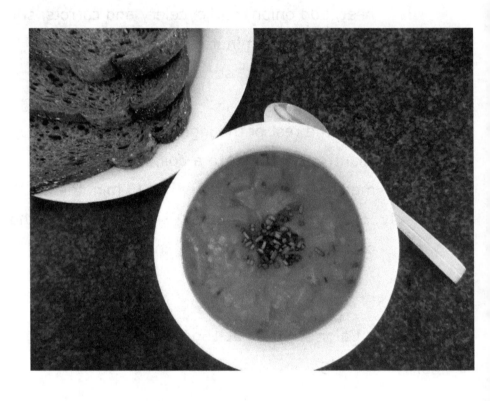

Lamb and Potato Stew

Preparation Time: 10 minutes

Cooking Time: 2 hours

Servings: 4

Ingredients:

- 2 and ½ lb. lamb shoulder, boneless and cut in small pieces
- Salt and black pepper to taste
- 1 yellow onion, chopped
- 3 tbsp. extra virgin olive oil
- 3 tomatoes, grated
- 1 and ½ cups chicken stock
- ½ cup dry white wine
- 1 bay leaf
- 2 and ½ lb. gold potatoes, cut into medium cubes
- ¾ cup green olives

Directions:

1. Heat a saucepan with the oil over medium high heat, add the lamb, brown for 10 minutes, transfer to a platter and keep warm for now.

2. Heat the pan again, add onion, stir and cook for 4 minutes.

3. Add tomatoes, stir, reduce heat to low and cook for 15 minutes.

4. Return lamb meat to pan, add wine and the rest of the ingredients except the potatoes and olives, stir, increase heat to medium high, bring to a boil, reduce heat again, cover pan and simmer for 30 minutes.

5. Add potatoes and olives, stir, cook for 1 more hour., divide into bowls and serve.

Nutrition: Calories 450, Fat 12gg, Fiber 4g, Carbs 33g, Protein 39g

Meatball and Pasta Soup

Preparation Time: 10 minutes

Cooking Time: 40 minutes

Servings: 4

Ingredients:

- 12 oz. pork meat, ground
- 12 oz. veal, ground
- Salt and black pepper to taste
- 1 garlic clove, minced
- 2 garlic cloves, sliced
- 2 tsp. thyme, chopped
- 1 egg, whisked
- 3 oz. Manchego, grated
- 2 tbsp. extra virgin olive oil
- 1/3 cup panko
- 4 cups chicken stock
- A pinch of saffron
- 15 oz. canned tomatoes, crushed
- 1 tbsp. parsley, chopped
- 8 oz. pasta

Directions:

1. In a bowl, mix veal with pork, 1 garlic clove, 1 tsp. thyme, ¼ tsp. paprika, salt, pepper to

taste, egg, manchego, panko, stir very well and shape medium meatballs out of this mix.

2. Heat a pan with 1 ½ tbsp. oil over medium high heat, add half of the meatballs, cook for 2 minutes on each side, transfer to paper towels, drain grease and put on a plate.

3. Repeat this with the rest of the meatballs.

4. Heat a saucepan with the rest of the oil, add sliced garlic, stir and cook for 1 minute.

5. Add the remaining ingredients and the meatballs, stir, reduce heat to medium low, cook for 25 minutes and season with salt and pepper.

6. Cook pasta according to instructions, drain, put in a bowl and mix with ½ cup soup.

7. Divide pasta into soup bowls, add soup and meatballs on top, sprinkle parsley all over and serve.

Nutrition: Calories 380, Fat 17gg, Fiber 2g, Carbs 28g, Protein 26g

Peas Soup

Preparation Time: 10 minutes

Cooking Time: 10 minutes

Servings: 4

Ingredients:

- 1 tsp. shallot, chopped
- 1 tbsp. butter
- 1-quart chicken stock
- 2 eggs
- 3 tbsp. lemon juice
- 2 cups peas
- 2 tbsp. parmesan, grated
- Salt and black pepper to taste

Directions:

1. Heat a saucepan with the butter over medium high heat, add shallot, stir and cook for 2 minutes.
2. Add stock, lemon juice, some salt and pepper and the whisked eggs .
3. Add more salt and pepper to taste, peas and parmesan cheese, stir, cook for 3 minutes, divide into bowls and serve.

Nutrition: Calories 180, Fat 39gg, Fiber 4g, Carbs 10g, Protein 14g

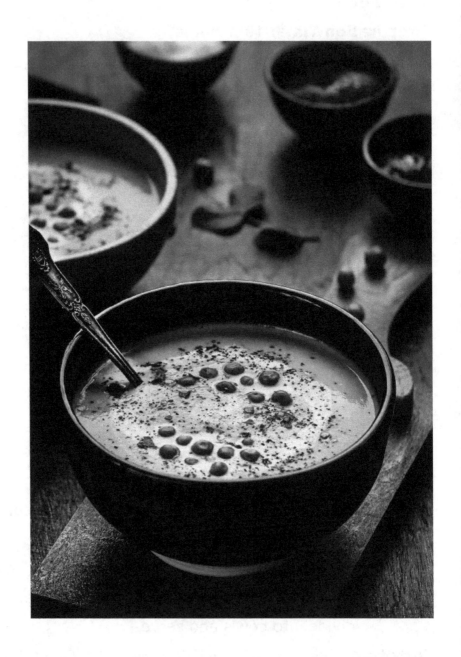

Minty Lamb Stew

Preparation Time: 10 minutes

Cooking Time: 1 hour and 45 minutes

Servings: 4

Ingredients:

- 3 cups orange juice
- ½ cup mint tea
- Salt and black pepper to taste
- 2 lb. lamb shoulder chops
- 1 tbsp. mustard, dry
- 3 tbsp. canola oil
- 1 tbsp. ras el hanout
- 1 carrot, chopped
- 1 yellow onion, chopped
- 1 celery rib, chopped
- 1 tbsp. ginger, grated
- 28 oz. canned tomatoes, crushed
- 1 tbsp. garlic, minced
- 2-star anise
- 1 cup apricots, dried and cut in halves
- 1 cinnamon stick
- ½ cup mint, chopped
- 15 oz. canned chickpeas, drained

- 6 tbsp. yogurt

Directions:

1. Put orange juice in a saucepan, bring to a boil over medium heat, take off heat, add tea leaves, cover and leave aside for 3 minutes, strain this and leave aside.

2. Heat a saucepan with 2 tbsp. oil over medium high heat, add lamb chops seasoned with salt, pepper, mustard and rasel hanout, toss, brown for 3 minutes on each side and transfer to a plate.

3. Add remaining oil to the saucepan, heat over medium heat, add ginger, onion, carrot, garlic and celery, stir and cook for 5 minutes.

4. Add orange juice, star anise, tomatoes, cinnamon stick, lamb, apricots, stir and cook for 1 hour and 30 minutes.

5. Transfer lamb chops to a cutting board, discard bones and chop.

6. Bring sauce from the pan to a boil, add chickpeas and mint, stir and cook for 10 minutes.

7. Discard cinnamon and star anise, divide into bowls and serve with yogurt on top.

Nutrition: Calories 560, Fat 24gg, Fiber 11g, Carbs 35g, Protein 33g

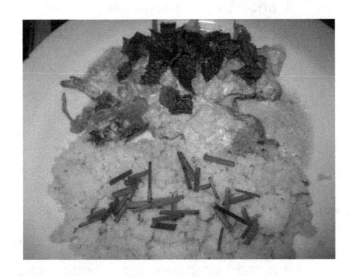

Spinach and Orzo Soup

Preparation Time: 10 minutes

Cooking Time: 10 minutes

Servings: 4

Ingredients:

- ½ cup orzo
- 6 cups chicken soup
- 1 and ½ cups parmesan, grated
- Salt and black pepper to taste
- 1 and ½ tsp. oregano, dried
- ¼ cup yellow onion, finely chopped
- 3 cups baby spinach
- 2 tbsp. lemon juice
- ½ cup peas, frozen

Directions:

1. Heat a saucepan with the stock over high heat, add oregano, orzo, onion, salt and pepper, stir, bring to a boil, cover and cook for 10 minutes.
2. Take soup off the heat, add salt and pepper to taste and the rest of the ingredients , stir well and divide into soup bowls. Serve right away.

Nutrition: Calories 201, Fat 5g, Fiber 3g, Carbs 28g, Protein 17g

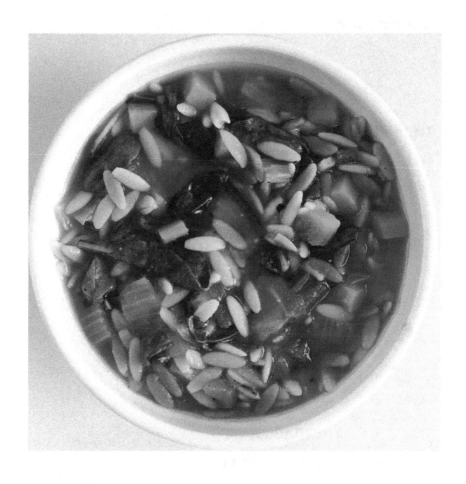

Minty Lentil and Spinach Soup

Preparation Time: 10 minutes

Cooking Time: 30 minutes

Servings: 6

Ingredients:

- 2 tbsp. olive oil
- 1 yellow onion, chopped
- A pinch of salt and black pepper
- 2 garlic cloves, minced
- 1 tsp. coriander, ground
- 1 tsp. cumin, ground
- 1 tsp. sumac
- 1 tsp. red pepper, crushed
- 2 tsp. mint, dried
- 1 tbsp. flour
- 6 cups veggie stock
- 3 cups water
- 12 oz. spinach, torn
- 1 and ½ cups brown lentils, rinsed

- 2 cups parsley, chopped
- Juice of 1 lime

Directions:

1. Heat up a pot with the oil over medium heat, add the onions, stir and sauté for 5 minutes.
2. Add garlic, salt, pepper, coriander, cumin, sumac, red pepper, mint and flour, stir and cook for another minute.
3. Add the stock, water and the other ingredients except the parsley and lime juice, stir, bring to a simmer and cook for 20 minutes.
4. Add the parsley and lime juice, cook the soup for 5 minutes more, ladle into bowls and serve.

Nutrition: Calories 170, Fat 7g, Fiber 6g, Carbs 22g, Protein 8g

Chicken and Apricots Stew

Preparation Time: 10 minutes

Cooking Time: 2 hours and 10 minutes

Servings: 4

Ingredients:

- 3 garlic cloves, minced
- 1 tbsp. parsley, chopped
- 20 saffron threads
- 3 tbsp. cilantro, chopped
- Salt and black pepper to taste
- 1 tsp. ginger, ground
- 2 tbsp. olive oil
- 3 red onions, thinly sliced
- 4 chicken drumsticks
- 5 oz. apricots, dried
- 2 tbsp. butter
- ¼ cup honey
- 2/3 cup walnuts, chopped
- ½ cinnamon stick

Directions:

1. Heat a pan over medium high heat, add saffron threads, toast them for 2 minutes, transfer to a bowl, cool down and crush.

2. Add the chicken pieces, 1 tbsp. cilantro, parsley, garlic, ginger, salt, pepper, oil and 2 tbsp. water, toss really well and keep in the fridge for 30 minutes.
3. Arrange onion on the bottom of a saucepan.
4. Add chicken and marinade, add 1 tbsp. butter, place on stove over medium high heat and cook for 15 minutes.
5. Add ¼ cup water, stir, cover pan, reduce heat to medium-low and simmer for 45 minutes.
6. Heat a pan over medium heat, add 2 tbsp. honey, cinnamon stick, apricots and ¾ cup water, stir, bring to a boil, reduce to low and simmer for 15 minutes.
7. Take off heat, discard cinnamon and leave to cool down.
8. Heat a pan with remaining butter over medium heat, add remaining honey and walnuts, stir, cook for 5 minutes and transfer to a plate.
9. Add chicken to apricot sauce, also season with salt, pepper and the rest of the cilantro

stir, cook for 10 minutes and serve on top of walnuts.

Nutrition: Calories 560, Fat 10g, Fiber 4g, Carbs 34g, Protein 44g

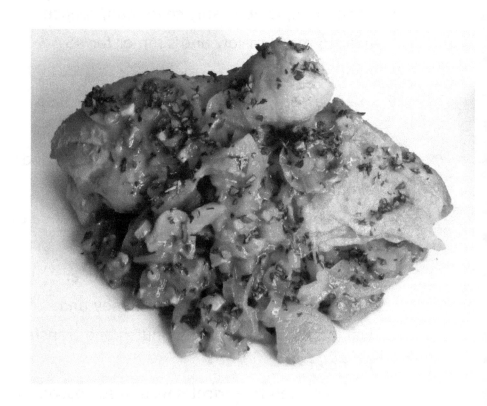

Fish and Veggie Stew

Preparation Time: 10 minutes

Cooking Time: 1 hour and 30 minutes

Servings: 4

Ingredients:

- 6 lemon wedges, pulp separated and chopped and some of the peel reserved
- 2 tbsp. parsley, chopped
- 2 tomatoes, cut in halves, peeled and grated
- 2 tbsp. cilantro, chopped
- 2 garlic cloves, minced
- ½ tsp. paprika
- 2 tbsp. water
- ½ cup water
- ½ tsp. cumin, ground
- Salt and black pepper to taste
- 4 bass fillets
- ¼ cup olive oil
- 3 carrots, sliced
- 1 red bell pepper, sliced lengthwise and thinly cut in strips
- 1 and ¼ lb. potatoes, peeled and sliced
- ½ cup olives

- 1 red onion, thinly sliced

Directions:

1. In a bowl, mix tomatoes with lemon pulp, cilantro, parsley, cumin, garlic, paprika, salt, pepper, 2 tbsp. water, 2 tsp. oil and the fish, toss to coat and keep in the fridge for 30 minutes.

2. Heat a saucepan with the water and some salt over medium high heat, add potatoes and carrots, stir, cook for 10 minutes and drain.

3. Heat a pan over medium heat, add bell pepper and ¼ cup water, cover, cook for 5 minutes and take off heat.

4. Coat a saucepan with remaining oil, add potatoes and carrots, ¼ cup water, onion slices, fish and its marinade, bell pepper strips, olives, salt and pepper, toss gently, cook for 45 minutes, divide into bowls and serve.

Nutrition: Calories 440, Fat 18g, Fiber 8g, Carbs 43g, Protein 30g

Tomato Soup

Preparation Time: 60 minutes

Cooking Time: 2 minutes

Servings: 4

Ingredients:

- ½ green bell pepper, chopped
- ½ red bell pepper, chopped
- 1 and ¾ lb. tomatoes, chopped
- ¼ cup bread, torn
- 9 tbsp. extra virgin olive oil
- 1 garlic clove, minced
- 2 tsp. sherry vinegar
- Salt and black pepper to taste
- 1 tbsp. cilantro, chopped
- A pinch of cumin, ground

Directions:

1. In a blender, mix green and red bell peppers with tomatoes, salt, pepper, 6 tbsp. oil, and the other ingredients except the bread and cilantro, and pulse well. Keep in the fridge for 1 hour.
2. Heat up a pan with remaining oil over medium high heat, add bread pieces, and toast them for 1 minute.
3. Divide cold soup into bowls, top with bread cubes and cilantro then serve.

Nutrition: Calories 260, Fat 23g, Fiber 2g, Carbs 11g, Protein 2g

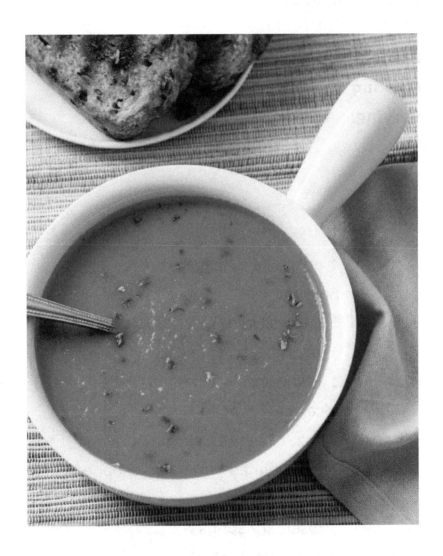

Chickpeas Soup

Preparation Time: 10 minutes

Cooking Time: 35 minutes

Servings: 4

Ingredients:

- 1 bunch kale, leaves torn
- Salt and black pepper to taste
- 3 tbsp. olive oil
- 1 celery stalk, chopped
- 1 yellow onion, chopped
- 1 carrot, chopped
- 30 oz. canned chickpeas, drained
- 14 oz. canned tomatoes, chopped
- 1 bay leaf
- 3 rosemary sprigs
- 4 cups veggie stock

Directions:

1. In a bowl, mix kale with half of the oil, salt and pepper, toss to coat., spread on a lined baking sheet, cook at 425°F for 12 minutes and leave aside to cool down.
2. Heat a saucepan with remaining oil over medium high heat, add carrot, celery, onion, some salt and pepper, stir and cook for 5 minutes.
3. Add the rest of the ingredients, toss and simmer for 20 minutes.
4. Discard rosemary and bay leaf, puree using a blender and divide into soup bowls. Top with roasted kale and serve.

Nutrition: Calories 360, Fat 14g, Fiber 11g, Carbs 53g, Protein 14g

Fish Soup

Preparation Time: 10 minutes
Cooking Time: 35 minutes
Servings: 6

Ingredients:

- 2 garlic cloves, minced
- 2 tbsp. olive oil
- 1 fennel bulb, sliced
- 1 yellow onion, chopped
- 1 pinch saffron, soaked in some orange juice for 10 minutes and drained
- 14 oz. canned tomatoes, peeled
- 1 strip orange zest
- 6 cups seafood stock
- 10 halibut fillet, cut into big pieces
- 20 shrimp, peeled and deveined
- 1 bunch parsley, chopped
- Salt and white pepper to taste

Directions:

1. Heat a saucepan with oil over medium high heat, add onion, garlic and fennel, stir and cook for 10 minutes.
2. Add saffron, tomatoes, orange zest and stock, stir, bring to a boil and simmer for 20 minutes.
3. Add fish and shrimp, stir and cook for 6 minutes..
4. Sprinkle parsley, salt and pepper, divide into bowls and serve.

Nutrition: Calories 340, Fat 20g, Fiber 3g, Carbs 23g, Protein 45g

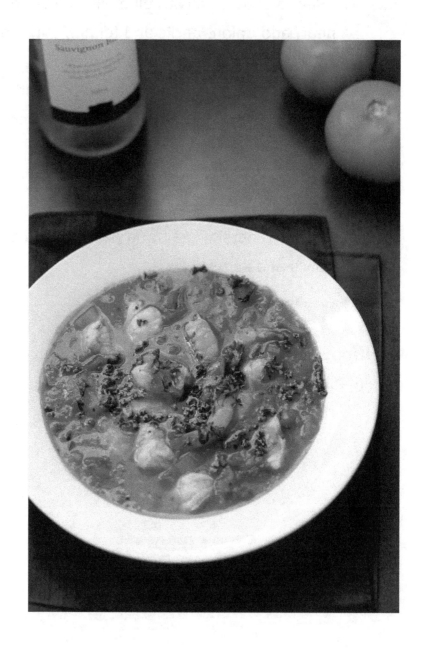

Chili Watermelon Soup

Preparation Time: 4 hours

Cooking Time: 5 minutes

Servings: 4

Ingredients:

- 3 lb. watermelon, sliced
- ½ tsp. chipotle chili powder
- 2 tbsp. olive oil
- Salt to taste
- 1 tomato, chopped
- 1 tbsp. shallot, chopped
- ¼ cup cilantro, chopped
- 1 small cucumber, chopped
- 1 small Serrano chili pepper, chopped
- 3 and ½ tbsp. lime juice
- ¼ cup crème Fraiche
- ½ tbsp. red wine vinegar

Directions:

1. In a bowl, mix 1 tbsp. oil with chipotle powder, stir and brush the watermelon with this mix.
2. Put the watermelon slices preheated grill pan over medium high heat, grill for 1 minute on each side, cool down, chop and put in a blender.
3. Add cucumber and the rest of the ingredients except the vinegar and the lime juice and pulse well.
4. Transfer to bowls, top with lime juice and vinegar, keep in the fridge for 4 hours and then serve.

Nutrition: Calories 115, Fat 0g, Fiber 2g, Carbs 18g, Protein 2g

Shrimp Soup

Preparation Time: 30 minutes

Cooking Time: 5 minutes

Servings: 6

Ingredients:

- 1 English cucumber, chopped
- 3 cups tomato juice
- 3 jarred roasted red peppers, chopped
- ½ cup olive oil
- 2 tbsp. sherry vinegar
- 1 tsp. sherry vinegar
- 1 garlic clove, mashed
- 2 baguette slices, cut into cubes and toasted
- Salt and black pepper to taste
- ½ tsp. cumin, ground
- ¾ lb. shrimp, peeled and deveined
- 1 tsp. thyme, chopped

Directions:

1. In a blender, mix cucumber with tomato juice, red peppers and pulse well, bread, 6 tbsp. oil, 2 tbsp. vinegar, cumin, salt, pepper and garlic, pulse again, transfer to a bowl and keep in the fridge for 30 minutes.
2. Heat a saucepan with 1 tbsp. oil over high heat, add shrimp, stir and cook for 2 minutes.
3. Add thyme, and the rest of the ingredients, cook for 1 minute and transfer to a plate. .
4. Divide cold soup into bowls, top with shrimp and serve. Enjoy!

Nutrition: Calories 230, Fat 7g, Fiber 10g, Carbs 24g, Protein 13g

Halibut and Veggies Stew

Preparation Time: 10 minutes

Cooking Time: 50 minutes

Servings: 4

Ingredients:

- 1 yellow onion, chopped
- 2 tbsp. oil
- 1 fennel bulb, stalks removed, sliced and roughly chopped
- 1 carrot, thinly sliced crosswise
- 1 red bell pepper, chopped
- 2 garlic cloves, minced
- 3 tbsp. tomato paste
- 16 oz. canned chickpeas, drained
- ½ cup dry white wine
- 1 tsp. thyme, chopped
- A pinch of smoked paprika
- Salt and black pepper to taste
- 1 bay leaf
- 2 pinches saffron
- 4 baguette slices, toasted
- 3 and ½ cups water
- 13 mussels, debearded

- 11 oz. halibut fillets, skinless and cut into chunks

Directions:

1. Heat a saucepan with the oil over medium high heat, add fennel, onion, bell pepper, garlic, tomato paste and carrot, stir and cook for 5 minutes. .

2. Add wine, stir and cook for 2 minutes. Add the rest of the ingredients except the halibut and mussels, stir, bring to a boil, cover and boil for 25 minutes.

3. Add, halibut and mussels, cover and simmer for 6 minutes more.

4. Discard unopened mussels, ladle into bowls and serve with toasted bread on the side.

Nutrition: Calories 450, Fat 12g, Fiber 13g, Carbs 47g, Protein 34g

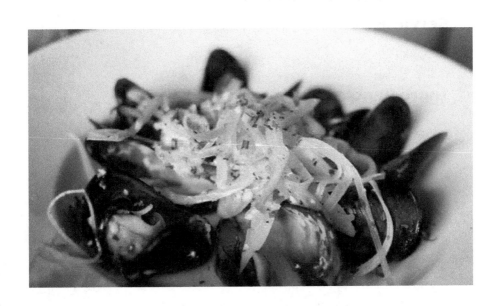

Cucumber Soup

Preparation Time: 10 minutes

Cooking Time: 6 minutes

Servings: 4

Ingredients:

- 3 bread slices
- ¼ cup almonds
- 4 tsp. almonds
- 3 cucumbers, peeled and chopped
- 3 garlic cloves, minced
- ½ cup warm water
- 6 scallions, thinly sliced
- ¼ cup white wine vinegar
- 3 tbsp. olive oil
- Salt to taste
- 1 tsp. lemon juice
- ½ cup green grapes, cut in halves

Directions:

1. Heat a pan over medium high heat, add almonds, stir, toast for 5 minutes, transfer to a plate and leave aside.
2. Soak bread in warm water for 2 minutes, transfer to a blender, add almost all the cucumber, salt, the oil, garlic, 5 scallions, lemon juice, vinegar and half of the almonds and pulse well.
3. Ladle soup into bowls, top with reserved ingredients and 2 tbsp. grapes and serve.

Nutrition: Calories 200, Fat 12g, Fiber 3g, Carbs 20g, Protein 6g

Chickpeas, Tomato and Kale Stew

Preparation Time: 10 minutes

Cooking Time: 30 minutes

Servings: 4

Ingredients:

- 1 yellow onion, chopped
- 1 tbsp. extra-virgin olive oil
- 2 cups sweet potatoes, peeled and chopped
- 1 ½ tsp. cumin, ground
- 4-inch cinnamon stick
- 14 oz. canned tomatoes, chopped
- 14 oz. canned chickpeas, drained
- 1 ½ tsp. honey
- 6 tbsp. orange juice
- 1 cup water
- Salt and black pepper to taste
- ½ cup green olives, pitted
- 2 cups kale leaves, chopped

Directions:

1. Heat a saucepan with the oil over medium high heat, add onion, cumin and cinnamon stir and cook for 5 minutes.
2. Add potatoes and the rest of the ingredients except the kale, stir, cover, reduce heat to medium-low and cook for 15 minutes.
3. Add kale , stir, cover again and cook for 10 minutes more. Divide into bowls and serve.

Nutrition: Calories 280, Fat 6g, Fiber 9g, Carbs 53g, Protein 10g

Veggie Stew

Preparation Time: 10 minutes

Cooking Time: 50 minutes

Servings: 4

Ingredients:

- 3 eggplants, chopped
- Salt and black pepper to taste
- 6 zucchinis, chopped
- 2 yellow onions, chopped
- 3 red bell peppers, chopped
- 56 oz. canned tomatoes, chopped
- A handful black olives, pitted and chopped
- A pinch of allspice, ground
- A pinch of cinnamon, ground
- 1 tsp. oregano, dried
- A drizzle of honey
- 1 tbsp. garbanzo bean flour mixed with 1 tbsp. water
- A drizzle of olive oil
- A pinch of red chili flakes
- 3 tbsp. Greek yogurt

Directions:

1. Heat a saucepan with the oil over medium high heat, add bell peppers, onions, some salt and pepper, stir and sauté for 4 minutes.
2. Add eggplant and the rest of the ingredients except the flour, olives, chili flakes and the yogurt, stir, bring to a boil, cover, reduce heat to medium-low and cook for 45 minutes.
3. Add the remaining ingredients except the yogurt, stir, cook for 1 minute, divide into bowls and serve with some Greek yogurt on top.

Nutrition: Calories 80, Fat 2g, Fiber 4g, Carbs 12g, Protein 3g

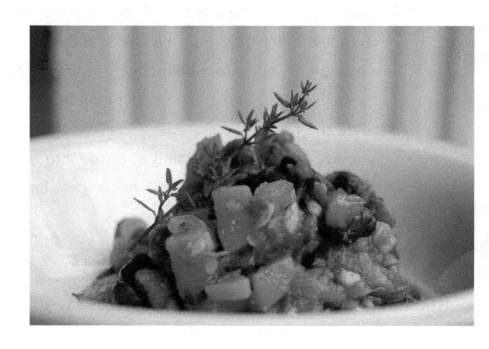

Beef and Eggplant Soup

Preparation Time: 10 minutes

Cooking Time: 30 minutes

Servings: 8

Ingredients:

- 1 yellow onion, chopped
- 1 tbsp. olive oil
- 1 garlic clove, minced
- 1 lb. beef, ground
- 1 lb. eggplant, chopped
- ¾ cup celery, chopped
- ¾ cup carrots, chopped
- Salt and black pepper to taste
- 29 oz. canned tomatoes, drained and chopped
- 28 oz. beef stock
- ½ tsp. nutmeg, ground
- ½ cup macaroni
- 2 tsp. parsley, chopped

- ½ cup parmesan cheese, grated

Directions:

1. Heat a large saucepan with the oil over medium heat, add onion, garlic and meat, stir and brown for 5 minutes..
2. Add celery, carrots and the other ingredients except the macaroni and the cheese, stir, bring to a simmer and cook for 20 minutes.
3. Add macaroni, stir and cook for 12 minutes.
4. Ladle into soup bowls, top with grated cheese and serve.

Nutrition: Calories 241, Fat 3g, Fiber 5g, Carbs 7g, Protein 10g

Melon Salad

Preparation Time: 10 minutes

Cooking Time: 20 Minutes

Servings: 6

Ingredients:

- ¼ tsp. Sea Salt
- ¼ tsp. Black Pepper
- 1 tbsp. Balsamic Vinegar
- 1 Cantaloupe, Quartered & Seeded
- 12 Watermelon, Small & Seedless
- 2 Cups Mozzarella Balls, Fresh
- 1/3 Cup Basil, Fresh & Torn
- 2 tbsp. Olive Oil

Directions:

1. Get out a melon baller and scoop out balls of cantaloupe, and the put them in a colander over a serving bowl.
2. Use your melon baller to cut the watermelon as well, and then put them in with your cantaloupe.

3. Allow your fruit to drain for ten minutes, and then refrigerate the juice for another recipe. It can even be added to smoothies.
4. Wipe the bowl dry, and then place your fruit in it.
5. Add in your basil, oil, vinegar, mozzarella and tomatoes before seasoning with salt and pepper.
6. Gently mix and serve immediately or chilled.

Nutrition:

Calories: 218

Protein: 10 g

Fat: 13 g

Carbs: 17 g

Orange Celery Salad

Preparation Time: 5 minutes

Cooking Time: 15 Minutes

Servings: 6

Ingredients:

- 1 tbsp. Lemon Juice, Fresh
- ¼ tsp. Sea Salt, Fine
- ¼ tsp. Black Pepper
- 1 tbsp. Olive Brine
- 1 tbsp. Olive Oil
- ¼ Cup Red Onion, Sliced
- ½ Cup Green Olives
- 2 Oranges, Peeled & Sliced
- 3 Celery Stalks, Sliced Diagonally in ½ Inch Slices

Directions:

1. Put your oranges, olives, onion and celery in a shallow bowl.
2. In a different bowl whisk your oil, olive brine and lemon juice, pour this over your salad.
3. Season with salt and pepper before serving.

Nutrition:

Calories: 65

Protein: 2 g

Fat: 0 g

Carbs: 9 g

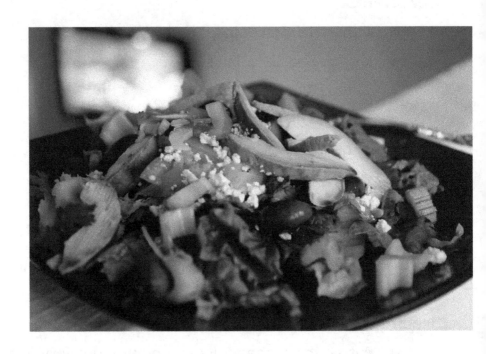

Roasted Broccoli Salad

Preparation Time: 30 Minutes

Cooking Time: 30 minutes

Servings: 4

Ingredients:

- 1 lb. Broccoli, Cut into Florets & Stem Sliced
- 3 tbsp. Olive Oil, Divided
- 1 Pint Cherry Tomatoes
- 1 ½ Teaspoons Honey, Raw & Divided
- 3 Cups Cubed Bread, Whole Grain
- 1 tbsp. Balsamic Vinegar
- ½ tsp. Black Pepper
- ¼ tsp. Sea Salt, Fine
- Grated Parmesan for Serving

Directions:

1. Start by heating your oven to 450, and then get out a rimmed baking sheet. Place it in the oven to heat up.
2. Drizzle your broccoli with a tbsp. of oil, and toss to coat.
3. Remove the baking sheet form the oven, and spoon the broccoli on it. Leave oil it eh bottom of the bowl and add in your tomatoes, toss to coat, and then toss your tomatoes with a tbsp.

of honey. Pour them on the same baking sheet as your broccoli.

4. Roast for fifteen minutes, and stir halfway through your cooking time.
5. Add in your bread, and then roast for three more minutes.
6. Whisk two tbsp. of oil, vinegar, and remaining honey. Season with salt and pepper. Pour this over your broccoli mix to serve.

Nutrition:

Calories: 226

Protein: 7 g

Fat: 12 g

Carbs: 26 g

Tomato Salad

Preparation Time: 5 minutes

Cooking Time: 20 Minutes

Servings: 4

Ingredients:

- 1 Cucumber, Sliced
- ¼ Cup Sun Dried Tomatoes, Chopped
- 1 lb. Tomatoes, Cubed
- ½ Cup Black Olives
- 1 Red Onion, Sliced
- 1 tbsp. Balsamic Vinegar
- ¼ Cup Parsley, Fresh & Chopped
- 2 tbsp. Olive Oil
- Sea Salt & Black Pepper to Taste

Directions:

1. Get out a bowl and combine all of your vegetables together. To make your dressing mix all your seasoning, olive oil and vinegar.
2. Toss with your salad and serve fresh.

Nutrition:

Calories: 126

Protein: 2.1 g

Fat: 9.2 g

Carbs: 11.5 g

Feta Beet Salad

Preparation Time: 5 minutes

Cooking Time: 5 Minutes

Servings: 4

Ingredients:

- 6 Red Beets, Cooked & Peeled
- 3 Oz. Feta Cheese, Cubed
- 2 tbsp. Olive Oil
- 2 tbsp. Balsamic Vinegar

Directions:

1. Combine everything together, and then serve.

Nutrition:

Calories: 230

Protein: 7.3 g

Fat: 12 g

Carbs: 26.3 g

Cauliflower & Tomato Salad

Preparation Time: 5 minutes

Time: 15 Minutes

Servings: 4

Ingredients:

- 1 Head Cauliflower, Chopped
- 2 tbsp. Parsley, Fresh & chopped
- 2 Cups Cherry Tomatoes, Halved
- 2 tbsp. Lemon Juice, Fresh
- 2 tbsp. Pine Nuts
- Sea Salt & Black Pepper to Taste

Directions:

1. Mix your lemon juice, cherry tomatoes, cauliflower and parsley together, and then season. Top with pine nuts, and mix well before serving.

Nutrition:

Calories: 64

Protein: 2.8 g

Fat: 3.3 g

Carbs: 7.9 g

Tuna Salad

Preparation Time: 10 minutes

Cooking Time: 0 minutes

Servings: 2

Ingredients:

- 12 oz. canned tuna in water, drained and flaked
- ¼ cup roasted red peppers, chopped
- 2 tbsp. capers, drained
- 8 kalamata olives, pitted and sliced
- 2 tbsp. olive oil
- 1 tbsp. parsley, chopped
- 1 tbsp. lemon juice
- A pinch of salt and black pepper

Directions:

3. In a bowl, combine the tuna with roasted peppers and the rest of the ingredients, toss, divide between plates and serve for breakfast.

Nutrition:

Calories 250,

Fat 17.5 g,

Fiber 0.6 g,

Carbs 2.6 g,

Protein 10.4 g

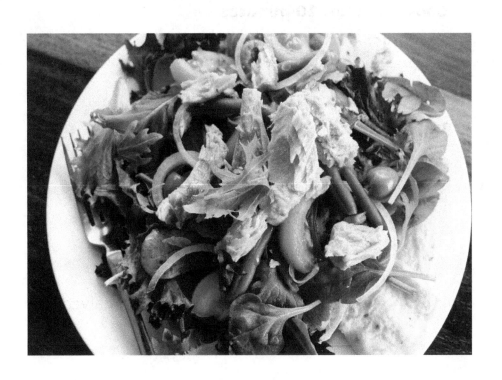

Corn and Shrimp Salad

Preparation Time: 10 minutes
Cooking Time: 10 minutes
Servings: 4

Ingredients:

- 4 ears of sweet corn, husked
- 1 avocado, peeled, pitted and chopped
- ½ cup basil, chopped
- A pinch of salt and black pepper
- 1 lb. shrimp, peeled and deveined
- 1 and ½ cups cherry tomatoes, halved
- ¼ cup olive oil

Directions:

1. Put the corn in a pot, add water to cover, bring to a boil over medium heat, cook for 6 minutes, drain, cool down, cut corn from the cob and put it in a bowl.

2. Thread the shrimp onto skewers and brush with some of the oil.
3. Place the skewers on the preheated grill, cook over medium heat for 2 minutes on each side, remove from skewers and add over the corn.
4. Add the rest of the ingredients to the bowl, toss, divide between plates and serve for breakfast.

Nutrition:

Calories 316,

Fat 22.5 g,

Fiber 5.6 g,

Carbs 23.6 g,

Protein 15.4 g

Tahini Spinach

Preparation Time: 5 minutes

Time: 5 Minutes

Servings: 4

Ingredients:

- 10 Spinach, Chopped
- ½ Cup Water
- 1 tbsp. Tahini
- 2 Cloves Garlic, Minced
- ¼ tsp. Cumin
- ¼ tsp. Paprika
- ¼ tsp. Cayenne Pepper
- 1/3 Cup Red Wine Vinegar
- Sea Salt & Black Pepper to Taste

Directions:

2. Add your spinach and water to the saucepan, and then boil it on high heat. Once boiling reduce to low, and cover. Allow it to cook on simmer for five minutes.

3. Add in your garlic, cumin, cayenne, red wine vinegar, paprika and tahini. Whisk well, and season with salt and pepper.

4. Drain your spinach and top with tahini sauce to serve.

Nutrition:

Calories: 69

Protein: 5 g

Fat: 3 g

Carbs: 8 g

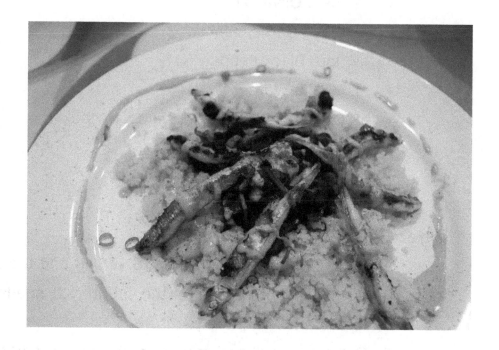

Asparagus Couscous

Preparation Time: 15 minutes

Cooking Time: 30 Minutes

Servings: 6

Ingredients :

- 1 Cup Goat Cheese, Garlic & Herb Flavored
- 1 ½ lbs. Asparagus, Trimmed & Chopped into 1 Inch Pieces
- 1 tbsp. Olive Oil
- 1 Clove Garlic, Minced
- ¼ tsp. Black Pepper
- 1 ¾ Cup Water
- 8 Oz. Whole Wheat Couscous, Uncooked
- ¼ tsp. Sea Salt, Fine

Directions:

1. Start by heating your oven to 425°F, and then put your goat cheese on the counter. It needs to come to room temperature.
2. Get out a bowl and mix your oil, pepper, garlic and asparagus. Spread the asparagus on a

baking sheet and roast for ten minutes. Make sure to stir at least once.

3. Remove it from the pan, and place your asparagus in a serving bowl.

4. Get out a medium saucepan, and bring your water to a boil. Add in your salt and couscous. Reduce the heat to medium-low, and then cover your saucepan. Cook for twelve minutes. All your water should be absorbed.

5. Pour the couscous in a bowl with asparagus, and ad din your goat cheese. Stir until melted, and serve warm.

Nutrition:

Calories: 263

Protein: 11 g

Fat: 9 g

Carbs: 36 g

Easy Spaghetti Squash

Preparation Time: 15 minutes

Cooking Time: 25 Minutes

Servings: 4

Ingredients:

- 2 Spring Onions, Chopped Fine
- 3 Cloves Garlic, Minced
- 1 Zucchini, Diced1 Red Bell Pepper, Diced
- 1 tbsp. Italian Seasoning
- 1 Tomato, Small & Chopped Fine
- 1 tbsp. Parsley, Fresh & Chopped
- Pinch Lemon Pepper
- Dash Sea Salt, Fine
- 4 Oz. Feta Cheese, Crumbled
- 3 Italian Sausage Links, Casing Removed
- 2 tbsp. Olive Oil
- 1 Spaghetti Sauce, Halved Lengthwise

Directions:

1. Start by heating your oven to 350°F, and get out a large baking sheet. Coat it with cooking spray, and then put your squash on it with the cut side down.
2. Bake at 350°F for forty-five minutes. It should be tender.

3. Turn the squash over, and bake for five more minutes. Scrape the strands into a larger bowl.

4. Heat up a tbsp. of olive oil in a skillet, and then add in your Italian sausage. Cook at eight minutes before removing it and placing it in a bowl.

5. Add another tbsp. of olive oil to the skillet and cook your garlic and onions until softened. This will take five minutes.

6. Throw in your Italian seasoning, red peppers and zucchini. Cook for another five minutes. Your vegetables should be softened.

7. Mix in your feta cheese and squash, cooking until the cheese has melted.

8. Stir in your sausage, and then season with lemon pepper and salt. Serve with parsley and tomato.

Nutrition:

Calories: 423

Protein: 18 g

Fat: 30 g

Carbs: 22 g

Garbanzo Bean Salad

Preparation Time: 10 minutes

Cooking Time: 0 minutes

Servings: 4

Ingredients:

- 1 and ½ cups cucumber, cubed
- 15 oz. canned garbanzo beans, drained and rinsed
- 3 oz. black olives, pitted and sliced
- 1 tomato, chopped
- ¼ cup red onion, chopped
- 5 cups salad greens
- A pinch of salt and black pepper
- ½ cup feta cheese, crumbled
- 3 tbsp. olive oil
- 1 tbsp. lemon juice
- ¼ cup parsley, chopped

Directions:

1. In a salad bowl, combine the garbanzo beans with the cucumber, tomato and the rest of the ingredients except the cheese and toss.
2. Divide the mix into small bowls, sprinkle the cheese on top and serve for breakfast.

Nutrition:

Calories 268,

Fat 16.5 g,

Fiber 7.6 g,

Carbs 36.6 g,

Protein 9.4 g

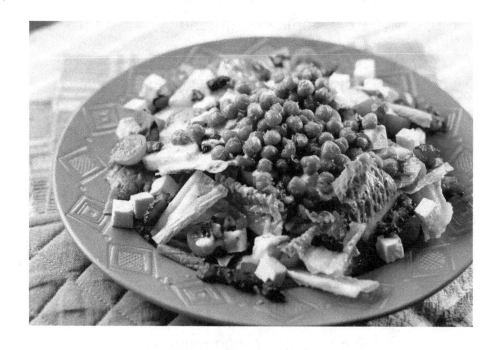

Spiced Chickpeas Bowls

Preparation Time: 10 minutes

Cooking Time: 30 minutes

Servings: 4

Ingredients :

- 15 oz. canned chickpeas, drained and rinsed
- ¼ tsp. cardamom, ground
- ½ tsp. cinnamon powder
- 1 and ½ tsp. turmeric powder
- 1 tsp. coriander, ground
- 1 tbsp. olive oil
- A pinch of salt and black pepper
- ¾ cup Greek yogurt
- ½ cup green olives, pitted and halved
- ½ cup cherry tomatoes, halved
- 1 cucumber, sliced

Directions:

1. Spread the chickpeas on a lined baking sheet, add the cardamom, cinnamon, turmeric, coriander, the oil, salt and pepper, toss and bake at 375°F for 30 minutes.
2. In a bowl, combine the roasted chickpeas with the rest of the ingredients, toss and serve for breakfast.

Nutrition:

Calories 519,

Fat 34.5 g,

Fiber 13.6 g,

Carbs 36.6 g,

Protein 11.4 g

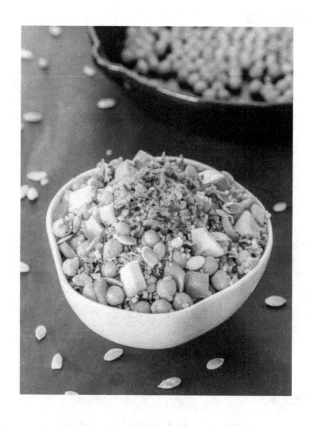

Tomato and Lentils Salad

Preparation Time: 10 minutes

Cooking Time: 35 minutes

Servings: 4

Ingredients:

- 2 yellow onions, chopped
- 4 garlic cloves, minced
- 2 cups brown lentils
- 1 tbsp. olive oil
- A pinch of salt and black pepper
- ½ tsp. sweet paprika
- ½ tsp. ginger, grated
- 3 cups water
- ¼ cup lemon juice
- ¾ cup Greek yogurt
- 3 tbsp. tomato paste

Directions:

1. Heat up a pot with the oil over medium-high heat, add the onions and sauté for 2 minutes.

2. Add the garlic and the lentils, stir and cook for 1 minute more.
3. Add the water, bring to a simmer and cook covered for 30 minutes.
4. Add the lemon juice and the remaining ingredients except the yogurt. Toss, divide the mix into bowls, top with the yogurt and serve.

Nutrition:

Calories 294,

Fat 3.5 g,

Fiber 9.6 g,

Carbs 26.6 g,

Protein 15.4 g

Egg and Arugula Salad

Preparation Time: 15 minutes

Cooking Time: 20 minutes

Servings: 4

Ingredients:

- 3 tomatoes
- 1 cucumber
- 4 eggs, boiled, peeled
- ½ cup black olives, pitted
- ¼ red onion, peeled
- ½ cup arugula
- 1/3 cup Plain yogurt
- 1 tsp. lemon juice
- ¼ tsp. paprika
- 1/3 tsp. Sea salt
- ½ tsp. dried oregano

Directions:

1. Chop tomatoes and cucumber into the medium cubes and transfer in the salad bowl.
2. Then tear arugula and add it in the salad bowl.

3. In the shallow bowl whisk together Plain yogurt, lemon juice, paprika, sea salt, and dried oregano.
4. Chop the boiled eggs roughly and add in the salad.
5. Add black olives (slice them if desired).
6. Then add red onion.
7. Shake the salad well.
8. Pour Plain yogurt dressing over the salad and stir it only before serving.

Nutrition:

Calories 169,

Fat 6.5 g,

Fiber 2.6 g,

Carbs 10.6 g,

Protein 9.4 g

Roasted Veggies

Preparation Time: 5 minutes

Cooking Time: 20 Minutes

Servings: 12

Ingredients :

- 6 Cloves Garlic
- 6 tbsp. Olive Oil
- 1 Fennel Bulb, Diced
- 1 Zucchini, Diced
- 2 Red Bell Peppers, Diced
- 6 Potatoes, Large & Diced
- 2 Teaspoons Sea Salt
- ½ Cup Balsamic Vinegar
- ¼ Cup Rosemary, Chopped & Fresh
- 2 Teaspoons Vegetable Bouillon Powder

Directions:

1. Start by heating your oven to 400°F.
2. Get out a baking dish and place your potatoes, fennel, zucchini, garlic and fennel on a baking dish, drizzling with olive oil.
3. Sprinkle with salt, bouillon powder, and rosemary. Mix well, and then bake at 450 for thirty to forty minutes. Mix your vinegar into the vegetables before serving.

Nutrition:

Calories: 675

Protein: 13 g

Fat: 21 g

Carbs: 112 g

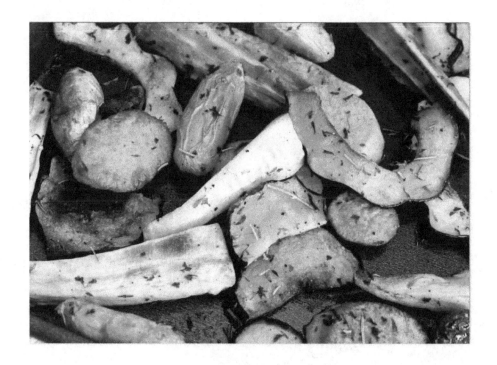

Roasted Eggplant Salad

Preparation Time: 15 minutes

Cooking Time: 40 Minutes

Servings: 6

Ingredients:

- 1 Red Onion, Sliced
- 2 tbsp. Parsley, Fresh & Chopped
- 1 tsp. Thyme
- 2 Cups Cherry Tomatoes, Halved
- Sea Salt & Black Pepper to Taste
- 1 tsp. Oregano
- 3 tbsp. Olive Oil
- 1 tsp. Basil
- 3 Eggplants, Peeled & Cubed

Directions:

1. Start by heating your oven to 350°F.
2. Season your eggplant with basil, salt, pepper, oregano, thyme and olive oil.
3. Spread it on a baking tray, and bake for a half hour.
4. Toss with your remaining ingredients before serving.

Nutrition:

Calories: 148

Protein: 3.5 g

Fat: 7.7 g

Carbs: 20.5 g

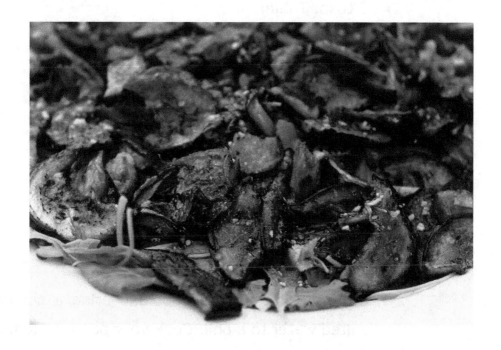

Penne with Tahini Sauce

Preparation Time: 10 minutes

Cooking Time: 20 Minutes

Servings: 8

Ingredients:

- 1/3 Cup Water
- 1 Cup Yogurt, Plain
- 1/8 Cup Lemon Juice
- 3 tbsp. Tahini
- 3 Cloves Garlic
- 1 Onion, Chopped
- ¼ Cup Olive Oil
- 2 Portobello Mushrooms, Large & Sliced
- ½ Red Bell Pepper, Diced
- 16 Oz. Penne Pasta
- ½ Cup Parsley, Fresh & Chopped
- Black Pepper to Taste

Directions:

1. Start by getting out a pot and bring a pot of salted water to a boil. Cook your pasta al dente per package instructions.
2. Mix your lemon juice and tahini together, and then place it tin a food processor. Process with garlic, water and yogurt. It should be smooth.

3. Get out a saucepan, and place it over medium heat. Heat up your oil, and cook your onions until soft.
4. Add in your mushroom and continue to cook until softened.
5. Add in your bell pepper, and cook until crispy.
6. Drain your pasta, and then toss with your tahini sauce, top with parsley and pepper and serve with vegetables.

Nutrition:

Calories: 332

Proteins: 11 g

Fat: 12 g

Carbs: 48 g

Parmesan Barley Risotto

Preparation Time: 15 minutes

Cooking Time: 30 Minutes

Servings: 6

Ingredients :

- 1 Cup yellow Onion, Chopped
- 1 tbsp. Olive Oil
- 4 Cups Vegetable Broth, Low Sodium
- 2 Cups Pearl Barley, Uncooked
- ½ Cup Dry White Wine
- 1 Cup Parmesan Cheese, Grated Fine & Divided
- Sea Salt & Black Pepper to Taste
- Fresh Chives, Chopped for Serving
- Lemon Wedges for Serving

Directions:

1. Add your broth into a saucepan and bring it to a simmer over medium-high heat.
2. Get out a stock pot and put it over medium-high heat as well. Heat up your oil before adding in your onion.

3. Cook for eight minutes and stir occasionally. Add in your barley and cook for two minutes more. Stir in your barley, cooking until it's toasted.
4. Pour in the wine, cooking for a minute more. Most of the liquid should have evaporated before adding in a cup of warm broth.
5. Cook and stir for two minutes. Your liquid should be absorbed. Add in the remaining broth by the cup, and cook until ach cup is absorbed fore adding more. It should take about two minutes each time. It will take a little longer for the last cup to be absorbed.
6. Remove from heat, and stir in a half a cup of cheese, and top with remaining cheese chives and lemon wedges.

Nutrition:

Calories; 346

Protein: 14 g

Fat: 7 g

Carbs: 56 g

Zucchini Pasta

Preparation Time: 15 minutes

Cooking Time: 30 Minutes

Servings: 4

Ingredients :

- 3 tbsp. Olive Oil
- 2 Cloves Garlic, Minced
- 3 Zucchini, Large & Diced
- Sea Salt & Black Pepper to Taste
- ½ Cup Milk, 2%
- ¼ tsp. Nutmeg
- 1 tbsp. Lemon Juice, Fresh
- ½ Cup Parmesan, Grated
- 8 Oz. Uncooked Farfalle Pasta

Directions:

1. Get out a skillet and place it over medium heat, and then heat up the oil. Add in your garlic and cook for a minute. Stir often so that it doesn't burn. Add in your salt, pepper and zucchini. Stir well, and cook covered for fifteen minutes. During this time, you'll want to stir the mixture twice.

2. Get out a microwave safe bowl, and heat the milk for thirty seconds. Stir in your nutmeg,

and then pour it into the skillet. Cook uncovered for five minutes. Stir occasionally to keep from burning.

3. Get out a stockpot and cook your pasta per package instructions. Drain the pasta, and then save two tbsp. of pasta water.

4. Stir everything together, and add in the cheese and lemon juice and pasta water.

Nutrition:

Calories: 410

Protein: 15 g

Fat: 17 g

Carbs: 45 g

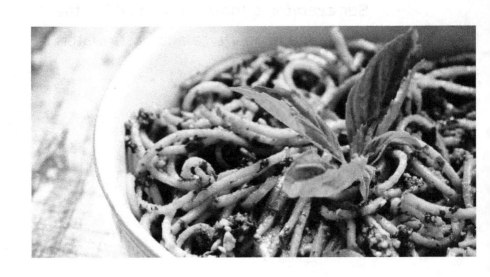

Quinoa and Eggs Salad

Preparation Time: 5 minutes

Cooking Time: 0 minutes

Servings: 4

Ingredients:

- 4 eggs, soft boiled, peeled and cut into wedges
- 2 cups baby arugula
- 2 cups cherry tomatoes, halved
- 1 cucumber, sliced
- 1 cup quinoa, cooked
- 1 cup almonds, chopped
- 1 avocado, peeled, pitted and sliced
- 1 tbsp. olive oil
- ½ cup mixed dill and mint, chopped
- A pinch of salt and black pepper
- Juice of 1 lemon

Directions:

3. In a large salad bowl, combine the eggs with the arugula and the rest of the ingredients, toss, divide between plates and serve for breakfast.

Nutrition:

Calories 519,

Fat 32.5 g,

Fiber 11.6 g,

Carbs 43.6 g,

Protein 19.4 g

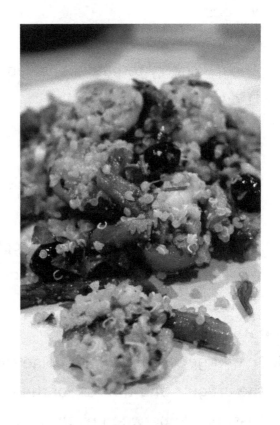

Feta & Spinach Pita Bake

Preparation Time: 10 minutes

Cooking Time: 20 Minutes

Servings: 6

Ingredients :

- 2 Roma Tomatoes, Chopped
- 6 Whole Wheat Pita Bread
- 1 Jar Sun Dried Tomato Pesto
- 4 Mushrooms, Fresh & Sliced
- 1 Bunch Spinach, Rinsed & Chopped
- 2 tbsp. Parmesan Cheese, Grated
- 3 tbsp. Olive Oil
- ½ Cup Feta Cheese, Crumbled
- Dash Black Pepper

Directions:

1. Start by heating the oven to 350°F, and get to your pita bread. Spread the tomato pesto

on the side of each one. Put them in a baking pan with the tomato side up.

2. Top with tomatoes, spinach, mushrooms, parmesan and feta. Drizzle with olive oil and season with pepper.

3. Bake for twelve minutes, and then serve cut into quarters.

Nutrition:

Calories; 350

Protein: 12 g

Fat: 17 g

Carbs: 42 g

Pistachio Arugula Salad

Preparation Time: 10 minutes

Cooking Time: 20 Minutes

Servings: 6

Ingredients :

- 6 Cups Kale, Chopped
- ¼ Cup Olive Oil
- 2 tbsp. Lemon Juice, Fresh
- ½ tsp. Smoked Paprika
- 2 Cups Arugula
- 1/3 Cup Pistachios, Unsalted & Shelled
- 6 tbsp. Parmesan Cheese, Grated

Directions:

1. Get out a salad bowl and combine your oil, lemon, smoked paprika and kale. Gently massage the leaves for half a minute. Your kale should be coated well.
2. Gently mix your arugula and pistachios when ready to serve.

Nutrition:

Calories: 150

Protein: 5 g

Fat: 12 g

Carbs: 8 g

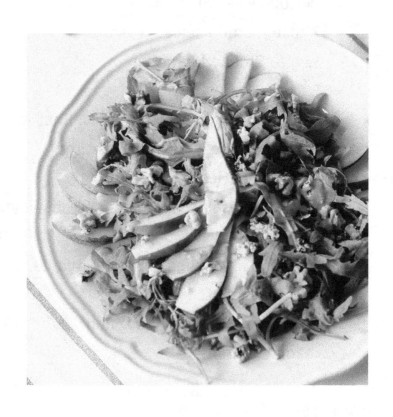

Easy Salad Wraps

Preparation Time: 10 minutes

Cooking Time: 20 Minutes

Servings: 4

Ingredients :

- 1 ½ Cups Cucumber, Seedless, Peeled & Chopped
- 1 Cup Tomato, Chopped
- ½ Cup Mint, Fresh & Chopped Fine
- Ounce Can Black Olives, Sliced & Drained
- ¼ Cup Red Onion, Diced
- 2 tbsp. olive Oil
- Sea Salt & Black Pepper to Taste
- 1 tbsp. Red Wine Vinegar
- ½ Cup Goat Cheese, Crumbled
- 4 Flatbread Wraps, Whole Wheat

Directions:

1. Get out a bowl and mix your tomato, mint, cucumber, onion and olives together.
2. Get out another bowl and whisk your vinegar, oil, pepper and salt. Drizzle this over your salad, and mix well.
3. Spread your goat cheese over the four wraps, and then spoon your salad filling in each one. Fold up to serve.

Nutrition:

Calories: 262

Protein: 7 g

Fat: 15 g

Carbs: 23 g

Margherita Slices

Preparation Time: 5 minutes

Cooking Time: 15 Minutes

Servings: 4

Ingredients :

- 1 Tomato, Cut into 8 Slices
- 1 Clove Garlic, Halved
- 1 tbsp. Olive Oil
- ¼ tsp. Oregano
- 1 Cup Mozzarella, Fresh & Sliced
- ¼ Cup Basil Leaves, Fresh, Tron & Lightly Packed
- Sea Salt & Black Pepper to Taste
- 2 Hoagie Rolls, 6 Inches Each

Directions:

1. Start by heating your oven broiler to high. Your rack should be four inches under the heating element.
2. Place the sliced bread on a rimmed baking sheet. Broil for a minute. Your bread should be

toasted lightly. Brush each one down with oil and rub your garlic over each half.

3.   Place the bread back on your baking sheet. Distribute the tomato slices on each one, and then sprinkle with oregano and cheese.

4.   Bake for one to two minutes, but check it after a minute. Your cheese should be melted.

5.   Top with basil and pepper before serving.

Nutrition:

Calories: 297

Protein: 12 g

Fat: 11 g

Carbs: 38 g

Vegetable Panini

Preparation Time: 15 minutes

Cooking Time: 25 Minutes

Servings: 4

Ingredients :

- 2 tbsp. Olive Oil, Divided
- ¼ Cup Onion, Diced
- 1 Cup Zucchini, Diced
- 1 ½ Cups Broccoli, Diced
- ¼ tsp. Oregano
- Sea Salt & Black Pepper to Taste
- 12 Oz. Jar Roasted Red Peppers, Drained & Chopped Fine
- 2 tbsp. Parmesan Cheese, Grated
- 1 Cup Mozzarella, Fresh & Sliced
- 2-Foot-Long Whole Grain Italian Loaf, Cut into 4 Pieces

Directions:

1. Heat your oven to 450°F, and then get out a baking sheet. Heat the oven with your baking sheet inside.

2. Get out a bowl and mix your broccoli, zucchini, oregano, pepper, onion and salt with a tbsp. of olive oil.
3. Remove your baking sheet from the oven and coat it in a nonstick cooking spray. Spread the vegetable mixture over it to roast for five minutes. Stir halfway through.
4. Remove it from the oven, and add your red pepper, and sprinkle with parmesan cheese. Mix everything together.
5. Get out a panini maker or grill pan, placing it over medium-high heat. Heat up a tbsp. of oil.
6. Spread the bread horizontally on it, but don't cut it all the way through. Fill with the vegetable mix, and then a slice of mozzarella cheese on top.
7. Close the sandwich and cook like you would a normal panini. With a press it should grill for five minutes. For a grill pan cook for two and a half minutes per side. Repeat for the remaining sandwiches.

Nutrition:

Calories: 352

Protein: 16 g

Fat: 15 g

Carbs: 45 g

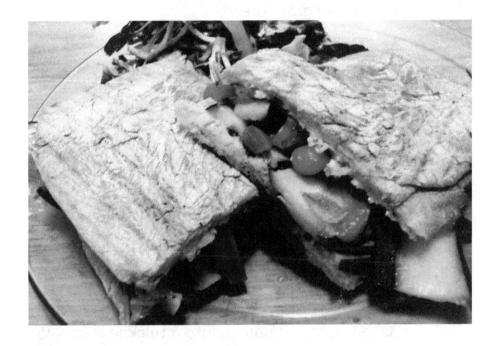

Baked Tomato

Preparation Time: 7 minutes

Cooking Time: 25 Minutes

Servings: 4

Ingredients :

- Whole grain bread
- Salt and pepper to taste
- 1 tbsp. of finely chopped basil
- 2 cloves of garlic. Finely chopped
- Extra virgin oil
- 2 large tomatoes

Directions:

1. Preheat your oven to 400°F.
2. Use the olive oil to brush the bottom of a baking dish. Set aside.
3. Slice the tomatoes into a thickness of a ½ inch. Lay the tomato pieces into the baking dish that you had prepared earlier. Sprinkle some basil and garlic on top of the tomatoes, season with pepper and salt to taste.

4. Then drizzle the slices of tomatoes with olive oil and then place the baking dish into the oven. Bake for about 20-25 minutes.

5. Remove from the oven, give it a few seconds to cool down and then serve and enjoy.

Tip: The tomato juice and olive oil at the bottom of the pan can be used as a dipping sauce. So if you want, you can put it into a small bowl and enjoy it with warm whole grain bread.

Nutrition:

Calories: 342

Protein: 16 g

Fat: 10 g

Carbs: 45 g

Mediterranean Humus Filled Roasted Veggies

Preparation Time: 7 minutes

Cooking Time: 25 Minutes

Servings: 12

Ingredients:

- 6 pitted kalamata olives quartered
- ½ cup (2oz.) of feta cheese
- 1 cup of hummus
- 2 tbsp. of olive oil
- 1 medium red bell pepper
- 1 small zucchini (6 inch)

Directions:

1. Heat a closed medium sized contact grill at 375°F for about 5 minutes.
2. Cut the summer squash and zucchini into half lengthwise. Use a spoon to scoop out the seeds from the two vegetables and discard the seeds.
3. Cut the red bell pepper around the stem and remove the stem and the seeds; cut them into quarters and set aside.
4. Use olive oil to brush the bell pepper, squash and zucchini pieces. Once done, place them on the grill. Do not close the grill.

5. Cook them for 4-6 minutes and turn only once. The vegetables should be tender by the end of the sixth minute. Remove from the grill and let them cool for 2 minutes. Cut the vegetables into 1-inch pieces.

6. Use a spoon to scoop 2 tbsp. of humus onto each piece of vegetable. Light drizzle the vegetables with cheese and top it with one piece of olive. Serve cold or warm.

Nutrition:

Calories: 342

Protein: 10 g

Fat: 15 g

Carbs: 35 g

Cucumber and Nuts Salad

Preparation Time: 20 minutes

Cooking Time: 3 hours

Servings: 10

Ingredients:

- ½ cup (2 oz.) of crumbled feta cheese
- 1/3 cup of chopped walnuts, toasted
- 1 chopped orange, peeled and sectioned
- ½ tsp. of salt
- 1 tbsp. of grated orange peel
- 1/3 cup of chopped fresh mint leaves that are loosely packed
- 1/3 cup of loosely packed flat-leafed chopped parsley
- ½ cup of sweetened dried cranberries
- ½ cup of chopped red onion
- ½ medium cucumber, unpeeled, seeded and chopped
- 2 tbsp. of olive oil
- ¼ cup of orange juice
- 1 cup of boiling water
- 1 cup of uncooked bulgur

Directions:

1. Start by placing the bulgur in a large heatproof bowl. Pour in some hot boiling water into the heatproof bowl and give the mixture a stir. Let the bulgur sit for about 1 hour or until the water has been absorbed.
2. Add in orange peel, mint, parsley, cranberries, onion, cucumber, salt, oil and orange juice and toss well. Cover the large bowl and refrigerate it for 2-3 hours or until the mixture is chilled.
3. Remove the mixture from the fridge and stir in some chopped oranges. Lightly sprinkle the mixture with cheese and walnuts. Serve and enjoy.

Nutrition:
Calories: 252
Protein: 16 g
Fat: 10 g
Carbs: 35 g

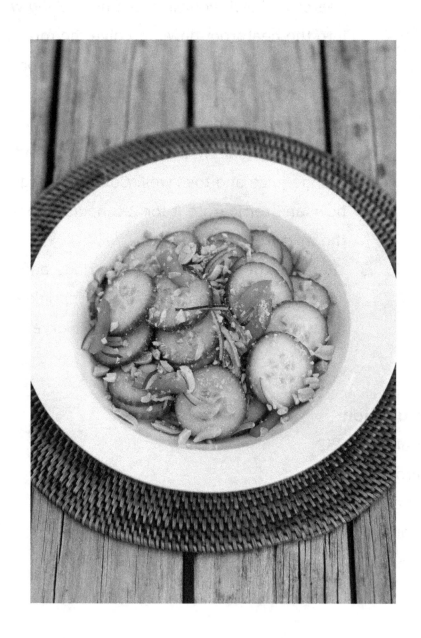